Melaleuca Essential Oil

Benefits, Properties, Applications, Studies & Recipes

by Ann Sullivan

Published in USA by:

Ann Sullivan
217 N. Seacrest Blvd #9
Boynton Beach
FL 33425

© Copyright 2015

ISBN-13: 978-1545129760
ISBN-10: 1545129762

TABLE OF CONTENTS

Introduction

What are essential oils, and how might they be used for therapeutic purposes?

First things first, essential oils are natural and organic. They are derived from the significant compounds found in the plants that possess them. Seeds, bark, flower petals, stems and roots, as well as other functional parts of the plant, can all be used to extract essential oils from a given plant. All of us have experienced the aromatic properties of the plants that provide essential oils, even if we are completely unaware of what was taking place when it happened. Remember the last time you bought, or received, a dozen roses? That beautiful aroma exploding from the roses, is just a part of the aromatic properties and qualities of the essential oils that can be extracted from that particular flower. In conjunction with providing specific smells to certain plant species, essential oils also offer plants a layer of protection against diseases and possible predators. They also have a significant role to perform in the pollination procedures of the associated plant species.

Essential oils are not water based. They are actually phytochemicals consisting of the powerful fragrant compounds of the plant. Phytochemicals are the compounds that occur naturally within the plant itself. This means that there are no synthetic additives, which are common in conventional medicines. Essential oils are fat soluble; however they do not possess the same fatty acids or lipids associated with animal or vegetable oil products. Essential oils are extremely clean, pure products that absorb into the skin almost immediately upon being touched. Essential oils are translucent when unadulterated and have a color range that spans from crystal clear to a deep and vibrant blue hue.

Here is an experiment you can try at home. Take a fresh lemon and slice it in half. Peel the rind from the fruit and squeeze it between your hands. That aromatic fruity smelling residue left behind is chock full of ingredients used to make essential oils.

Essential oils should not be confused with fragrance producing oils or perfumes. Essential oils are natural and organic and are taken directly from the plant. Perfumes and fragrance oils are either artificially created, or manufactured with synthetic solutions and do not possess the same therapeutic properties as essential oils. Essential oils are super concentrated substances, which means that a very little, usually a drop or two, will go a long way. The aromas and chemical compounds associated with essential oils allow them to provide therapeutic benefits for both physical and psychological procedures.

Essential oils are offered by a number of manufacturers and distributors around the world. They vary in price and quality, which is determined by a number of different factors. The country of origin for the plant species being used, how rare the botanical is, how much oil can be produced by a specific plant, growing climate present for the plants, and standards applied by the distiller/manufacturer, will all play a very important role in determining price and effectiveness of the essential oils being produced.

Essential oils are generally sold in small bottles or vials separately, or in slightly larger containers consisting of essential oil blends. The benefit of buying blends is that you can eliminate the need to purchase all essential oils separately. The disadvantage of buying blends is that you have no control of the mixture.

Chapter 3 will further detail past scientific research on melaleuca essential oil.

Now, let's get down to it – **Essential Oil 101: the Basics of Melaleuca.**

Summary: Melaleuca, or Melaleuca alternifolia, is also known as tea tree oil or snake oil, and has been used to effectively strengthen the body's natural defenses against skin conditions, as well as provide support to the immune system. This extremely popular oil has enormous benefits and is cultivated all over the world, from Guatemala to France, from the US to Australia to China. The melaleuca species grows best in swampland and has two chemotypes, both of which are composed of terpinen-4-ol or terpinenol-4, the components that make the oil so versatile.

Description: Melaleuca oil is commonly extracted through steam distillation. The leaves are most often used.

The oil is clear yellow in color, thin in consistency, and has a medium earthy and woody scent.

Uses: Beyond those applications previously mentioned, additional uses for melaleuca essential oil include supporting the body's natural defenses against colds, flu, skin issues, herpes, yeast infection, athlete's foot, acne, candida, chicken pox, corns, itching, spots, sores, warts, oily skin, ringworm, sinusitis, urethritis, whooping cough, migraine, insect bites, cuts, wounds, cold sores, and gum issues. Melaleuca also strengthens the immune system and can serve as a disinfectant. When it comes to mood and emotion, melaleuca can help one feel cleansed and refreshed.

Properties: Immune stimulant, antiviral, antifungal, antibacterial, antibiotic, anti-inflammatory, disinfectant and astringent.

Application: Dilute 1:1 with a carrier oil. You can apply topically, inhale directly, diffuse or use as a dietary supplement.

Safety Precautions: Melaleuca has been approved by the FDA for internal consumption and so can be used as a dietary supplement. However, if pregnant, breastfeeding or diabetic, consult a physician before using this oil. Repeat usage may cause contact sensitization.

Fun facts: Melaleuca is so named, because it was derived from the Greek words for "black" and "white," which are "melas" and "leukos," due to the dark leaves and the white bark of the tree.

The other names for melaleuca – tea tree oil and snake oil – also have interesting histories. Captain Cook actually named the melaleuca "tea tree" in 1770 after arriving in Botany Bay, Australia and discovering that the leaves from this tree made for delicious tea. Thereafter, the tea served as a therapeutic aid for the European settlers.

As for the term "snake oil," there are two stories in regards to its origination. The first is that melaleuca was used by the Australian aborigines to treat snake bites. Being that Australia has more than 100 species of the world's most venomous snakes, it's no wonder that they'd find this purpose for melaleuca.

A second story is that when America was settled, this oil was high in demand. So many a salesman materialized and began passing off melaleuca of tainted quality. These slick salesmen were referred to as Snake Oil Salesmen

Chapter 1:
Benefits of Melaleuca Essential Oil

Melaleuca oil offers a number of therapeutic benefits; but you may be wondering what these benefits are. In this chapter, we'll take a closer look at the history of melaleuca and its many uses.

Cultivation of Melaleuca

Melaleuca is of the Myrtaceae, the myrtle family of plants native to Australia. With over 200 species, melaleuca is largely touted for its cleansing and soothing abilities. The trees grow in the woodland, shrubland, or open forest, often near waterways or swamps. When cultivated, they are popularly harvested in gardens in Australia and other tropical areas. Depending on the species, melaleuca trees or shrubs can grow anywhere from 6-98 feet tall. Larger species are also called tea trees, while smaller species are often referred to as honey myrtles. Some species shed their bark in sheets, and these are known as paperbarks. All species have a flaky bark and evergreen leaves, and they often produce flowers of various colors – red, white, pink, yellow or green – which are densely clustered. The fruit that these trees produce is small and contains dozens of seeds.

Native to the Northeast coast of New South Wales and to Southeast Queensland in Australia, Melaleuca alternifolia is the primary species used in the making of tea tree essential oil, due to its antibiotic and antifungal properties. The oil is yellow or clear and exudes a fresh camphorous scent.

A History of Melaleuca

For centuries, the Aborigines of Australia have used melaleuca leaves for their therapeutic qualities. They would often chew the premature leaves in order to relieve headaches and also utilized their healing properties to treat a litany of ailments. Combined with clay, melaleuca was applied to skin to treat skin conditions or infections. The Aborigines even cleansed themselves in the water beneath melaleuca trees, because they believed it was healing.

It wasn't until 1922 that the properties of Melaleuca alternifolia became more widely known to the outside world. Arthur Penfold, an Australian chemist from the Sydney Museum of Technology and Applied Science, led a team to study the oil. They distilled melaleuca and found that it had intense antifungal and antibacterial properties. The oil was then touted globally as a powerful germicide which attacked intrusive germs, without harming normal skin cells. For a long time, melaleuca was an incredibly popular treatment for all kinds of infections and maladies, from ulcers to thrush, from head lice to ringworm, from gingivitis to tonsillitis. The oil was used by dentists, doctors, and even vets.

With World War II came the rapid rise and then decline of melaleuca essential oil. Because it was so popular, it was used in battle to disinfect war wounds and, thus, supply dwindled so far that it could no longer meet the demand; thus, melaleuca was no longer a cheap commodity. Manufacturers turned to other cheaper alternatives to fill the demand, which led to a decline in the melaleuca industry. The oil and its value was nearly abandoned.

However, the 60's brought melaleuca back to life, as new research uncovered its more than 100 components and revealed its heretofore undiscovered capacity in supporting the body's natural defenses against gynecological infections, foot issues, boils, and many other ailments. These newfound discoveries resurrected the oil and it grew commercially.

In the 90's and presently, considerable research has been done and is ongoing in relation to this powerful oil, its properties, and its potential. Papers and reviews regularly validate melaleuca's effectiveness in healing and discover new valuable uses to put the oil to. In the 90's, an Australian research team, led by Associate Professor Tom Riley from the University of Western Australia, revealed the oil's impact on MSRA (methicillin-resistant Staphylococcus aureus), a hospital bug that had mutated to the point that it was resistant to nearly all synthetic antibiotics. MSRA is prevalent in those with skin lesions, particularly when coupled with low immune systems or wounds following an operation. Being that MSRA is contagious, it transferred through hospital staff from patient to patient and had grown from infecting 3% in the 80's to 40% in the late 90's. When introduced into hospital settings, melaleuca essential oil served as an effective disinfectant for the resistant bacteria.

Chemical Components

In order to generate the essential oil from the tree, the leaves must be steam distilled. This results in the oil's key chemical components. With more than 98 compounds, melaleuca's primary chemicals are the anti-inflammatory and antimicrobial terpinen-4-ol chemotype. The oil also contains a terpinolene chemotype and four 1,8-cineole chemotypes. Any adverse reactions or allergies to tea tree oil is likely due to one of the 1,8-cineole chemotypes.

Main Properties of Melaleuca Essential Oil

Along with the properties previously mentioned in the introduction, melaleuca oil possesses immunostimulant, antiviral, antifungal, antibacterial, antibiotic, anti-inflammatory, disinfectant and astringent. With such a versatile range, melaleuca is well equipped to fight off any pathogen in the body's path and is a necessary addition to any essential oils kit.

Melaleuca, as mentioned, is composed of many natural chemicals, among them terpinen-4-ol. These components are what instill the enormously beneficial properties within melaleuca essential oil. We'll outline these properties below.

Disinfectant & Cleaner

As in the case of MSRA, melaleuca can be added to household cleaners to disinfect your home. As a cleaning agent, melaleuca eliminates contamination, which means your household will be healthier, on the whole, becoming sick less often. Melaleuca can be used to clean dishes, clothing, and practically any surface.

Antioxidant

Anything high in antioxidants – whether fruit, beans, or essential oils – is a powerful advocate for your body. Antioxidants both protect against free radicals and repair their damage. What are free radicals? Free radicals are destructive chemicals that invade your body, produced by substances both inside and out. Some free radicals (or oxidants) form through normal bodily reactions, like inflammation, metabolism and aerobic respiration. Other free radicals form outside the body, but enter it due to exposure. These include harmful pollutants, toxins, smoking, drinking alcohol, X-rays, and UV rays, to name a few. Although our bodies produce their own antioxidants, these often become damaged as we grow older; thus, introducing antioxidants into our bodies via essential oils allows these nutrients and enzymes to assist in chemical reactions which destroy the oxidants or free radicals. Melaleuca essential oil is a moderate antioxidant, aiming to detox the body of free radicals that lead to disease.

Antibacterial

Melaleuca's antibacterial properties make it a powerful protectant against diseases produced by bacteria, such as skin issues and infections. What's great is that, unlike some prescription drugs, melaleuca has no ill effects on body wellness or on the healthy natural flora that exists within the stomach and intestines. You can read about melaleuca's antibacterial properties here and here.

Antifungal

While bacteria and viruses are plenty evil, fungi commonly lead to the most deadly infections, whether external or internal. Your ears, throat and nose are the most likely to become infected by fungi, the infections of which can be both excruciating and unsightly. If left untreated, fungal infections can kill, as they may spread to the brain. Melaleuca essential oil protects against these infections and more.

Antiviral

The antiviral protection that melaleuca essential oil grants will empower the immune system at its core, building up a tougher wall of security that most colds, measles or mumps are unlikely to scale. By boosting white blood cell count and function, this immune stimulant will ensure that your body is better prepared to protect against deadly viral infections.

Anti-inflammatory

External or internal inflammation can be reduced through the use of melaleuca essential oil. For instance, if you or your patient has swollen fingers from arthritis or a swollen knee from a sport's injury, oral application of melaleuca essential oil may decrease irritation or redness, while also soothing the pain that accompanies inflammation. To learn more about melaleuca's anti-inflammatory properties, read this study.

Astringent

Astringents are chemical compounds that shrink body tissues, which means they can aid skin issues and irritations, everything from acne to insect bites. The astringent property of melaleuca essential oil benefits everything from skin to hair to gums to muscles to intestines. As an astringent, melaleuca is an anti-agent, combating muscle loss through the ability to strengthen.

Common Therapeutic Uses

Melaleuca has traditionally been used for its soothing and healing properties and, as an antioxidant with the primary chemical of terpinen-4-ol, melaleuca essential oil is particularly helpful when it comes to fighting inflammation and bacteria. The highly concentrated oil serves as a tonic which may be used to support the immune system. Let's take a look at some of the oil's primary therapeutic uses.

Skin Care

Melaleuca essential oil can be used both to protect against infections, heal and maintain your skin's tone and condition. The oil is a topical antiseptic and, as mentioned, has been shown to effectively eliminate the staph bacteria, MRSA; thus, it can protect against infections in wounds, as well as in burns and blisters. As you may have guessed, it can also be used to support the body's natural defenses against skin issues like acne. Though the results may come more slowly than, say, benzoyl peroxide, the application is not damaging to your skin's overall wellness. The antimicrobial terpenes work to cleanse your skin naturally. Moreover, melaleuca can target fungal infections, such as ringworm, which can be highly contagious. Inhibiting the spread of fungal infection is crucial to your overall wellness. Read about the role melaleuca can play in skin disease here.

Hair & Scalp

If you have unhealthy hair or dandruff, melaleuca is just what you need to give your hair's wellness a boost, while eliminating flaky and itchy scalp. As opposed to the harsh, dry, damaging chemicals in dandruff shampoos, melaleuca is a therapeutic supplement that serves your skin and hair naturally. Melaleuca can also be used to eliminate head lice and other parasites and is particularly effective when combined with peppermint essential oil.

Oral Health

The antiseptic properties in melaleuca mean that the oil's components are active in strengthening the body's natural defenses against oral fungal or bacterial infections. Used as a mouth rinse, melaleuca kills bad breath bacteria and also eliminates plaque. It also reduces gum bleeding, and maintains the mouth's overall wellness and cleanliness. Toothpaste, mouthwash, and many other oral wellness products contain melaleuca for this reason. Note: unless your tea tree oil is of high-quality, therapeutic grade and certified to be taken internally, do not swallow. The compounds can be toxic, leading to disorientation, nausea, and even coma.

Sore Throat

Melaleuca eliminates the bacteria in the tonsils and throat which causes sore throat and other throat issues. An oral dosage of tea tree oil will soothe the throat, while an aromatic dosage will clear congestion of the chest and sinuses. Again, do not swallow tea tree oil unless your brand's label declares it safe to do so.

Insect Stings & Bites

Because melaleuca is such an effective disinfectant and also possesses properties that both relieve pain and help eliminate itching, the oil is a surefire solution for insect stings and bites. With a little dab on the wound, topical application of tea tree oil can bring faster relief and healing. Melaleuca also staves off insects in the first place. A couple studies on the insecticidal properties of melaleuca can be found here and here.

Fungal Infections

Skin fungal infections, such as athlete's foot, dermatitis, and eczema, can all be relieved with melaleuca oil, due to the oil's impressive antifungal properties. The oil can be particularly effective when it comes to insidious nail infections. Melaleuca combats nail infections at their core, eliminating the fungus that produces the unsightly infection, as well as relieving any uncomfortable symptoms associated with the infection.

Household Cleaner

Melaleuca can either be used on its own or added to household cleaners to disinfect your home. As a cleaning agent, melaleuca eliminates contamination, which means your household will be healthier, on the whole, falling ill less often. As mentioned previously, melaleuca can be used to clean dishes, clothing, and practically any surface.

Immune System

Melaleuca is a superb immune system support which boosts circulation and increases white blood cell count. By doing so, this immune stimulant will ensure that your body is better prepared to protect against deadly viral infections. Research has been done on the benefits of melaleuca when it comes to the immune system; one study examining the oil's effects on influenza can be found here.

Safety Precautions & Common Applications

Safety

Some adverse effects may evolve when using pure essential oils. Some essential oils should not be used when pregnant, for example, as they may cause miscarriage. Allergic reactions, too, may occur, especially when applied topically. Always administer an allergy test before committing fully to topical application. When used with other medications, essential oils may react negatively. If you are on any current prescription medications or have a chronic illness, such as high blood pressure, epilepsy or liver disease, then researching the effects of essential oils against your own personal medical history will eliminate any potentially problematic issues.

Melaleuca has been approved by the FDA for internal consumption and so can be used as a dietary supplement. However, unless your tea tree oil is of high-quality, therapeutic grade, and certified to be taken internally, it is advised not to take the oil orally. The compounds can be toxic, leading to disorientation, nausea, and even coma. If pregnant, breastfeeding or diabetic, consult a physician before using this oil. Repeat usage may cause contact sensitization.

Blends

Oftentimes, essential oils are manufactured as blends of several pure oils. For instance, the Protective Oil Blend is a mix of cinnamon, clove, rosemary, and eucalyptus. This blend can be used to boost the immune system to help support the body's defenses against colds, viruses and flus. The downside to blends is that the more oils added to the mix, the higher the probability your patient may react negatively to the blend if he/she is prone to allergies. There is also the possibility of phototoxicity when working with blends.

Regardless of these possible effects, essential oils are a

viable option for support the body's defenses against a number of conditions. Those looking to enhance the maintenance of their own personal wellness, or that of their families, should become educated on the uses of essential oils, their natural remedies and the methods of application. Only then can you begin building your kit of essential oils for survival.

Chapter 2:
Recipes for Melaleuca Essential Oil

In this chapter, we'll offer various recipes for melaleuca essential oil, both for pure melaleuca supportive remedies and for blends which incorporate the oil. For pure supportive remedies, we've provided the appropriate application and dosage to target specific ailments, from acne to sinus infections. When it comes to blends, herbalists and aromatherapists often combine melaleuca essential oil with clary sage, cinnamon, clove, lavender, geranium, lemon, rosemary, thyme, myrrh, and rosewood. We'll offer some fantastic supportive blending options in the second half of this chapter.

Pure Supportive Remedies

Acne

Target acne with a single drop of tea tree oil. Dab onto acne breakouts or simply place a drop into your natural cleanser.

Allergies

Relieve allergies by diluting tea tree essential oil in a 1:1 ratio with a carrier oil and apply topically, massaging the oil into the abdomen, chest and the reflex points of the feet.

Aneurysm

Help protect against aneurysm by steaming two drops of tea tree essential oil in a pan of water. Then remove the steaming pan from the stove, pour into a bowl, place a towel over your head and inhale. If you don't feel it's done its job the first time, you can reheat that same water and use it once more without adding more oil. You can also simply inhale directly or massage the oil into the soles of your feet.

Athlete's Foot

Dilute melaleuca essential oil in a 1:1 ratio with a carrier oil and massage into your feet. You can also add two drops of tea tree to a sea salt foot bath or soak a pair of socks in warm water with two drops of tea tree and wear them for a half hour. Place one drop in shoes to rid of contact fungus for extended support.

Bacterial Infections

Combat bacterial infections by diluting tea tree essential oil in a 1:1 ratio with a carrier oil and applying topically over the affected area or massaging into the reflex points of the feet. You may also place a few drops in a bath or diffuse the oil for a similar effect.

Boils

Target boils by diluting tea tree essential oil in a 1:1 ratio with a carrier oil and applying topically over the affected area.

Bronchitis

For a great bronchitis remedy, dilute melaleuca essential oil in a 1:1 ratio with a carrier oil, then apply topically, massaging into the throat, chest, back and the reflex points of the feet. You may also steam two drops of tea tree essential oil in a pan of water, remove the steaming pan from the stove, pour into a bowl, place a towel over your head and inhale. If you don't feel it's done its job the first time, you can reheat that same water and use it once more without adding more oil. For an all-day solution, place a drop of oil onto your shirt collar or inhale directly.

Candida

Eliminate candida by diluting melaleuca essential oil with a carrier oil and massaging over affected area. You can also take tea tree orally (*make sure it's therapeutic grade), through use in a capsule or as a food additive.

Canker Sores

Relieve canker sores by diluting tea tree essential oil with a carrier oil and dabbing onto the sore 1-3 times daily, until the sore disappears.

Cavities

Protect against cavities by adding a drop of tea tree oil to your toothbrush before you apply toothpaste. You can also add a drop afterwards to disinfect your brush.

Chicken Pox

Combat chickenpox by diffusing tea tree essential oil in the area of the infected patient. You can also apply topically, diluting 3-4 drops tea tree oil per teaspoon of coconut oil and applying over the pox. You may dilute further for sensitive skin or small children.

Cold Sores

To eliminate or stave off cold sores, dilute tea tree essential oil in a 1:1 ratio with a carrier oil and dab directly onto the cold sore or apply as a lip balm.

Colds

Combat colds by diffusing tea tree essential oil throughout the home or place several drops in your wet laundry before drying. If you prefer inhalation therapy, steam two drops of tea tree essential oil in a pan of water, remove the steaming pan from the stove, pour into a bowl, place a towel over your head and inhale. You can also apply topically by diluting tea tree essential oil in a 1:1 ratio with a carrier oil and massaging into the chest and the soles of the feet.

Coughs

See above application for colds; same can be used for coughs.

Cuts

To accelerate skin repair and soothe pain, dilute melaleuca essential oil in a 1:1 ratio with a carrier oil and apply topically to the affected area.

Dermatitis

Dermatitis and other skin inflammation issues can be targeted by diluting melaleuca essential oil in a 1:1 ratio with a carrier oil and applying topically to the affected area.

Dry/Itchy Eyes

Combat dry, itchy eyes by diluting tea tree essential oil

or steaming two drops in a pan of water, removing the steaming pan from the stove, pouring it into a bowl, placing a towel over your head and inhaling.

Ear Infection/Ache

Relieve earaches or infections by diluting 1 drop of tea tree oil in 1-2 TB of water. Using a dropper, place one drop of the combo into the ear for 30-60 seconds.

Eczema

Support the body's natural defenses against eczema by diluting melaleuca essential oil in a 1:1 ratio with a carrier oil and applying topically to the affected area.

Flu

Strengthen the immune system against the flu according to its symptoms by diluting melaleuca essential oil in a 1:1 ratio with a carrier oil, then apply topically, massaging it into sore muscles and joints, into the reflex points of the feet, or over the abdominal area, if you're experiencing diarrhea. You can also diffuse throughout the home to support general wellness during cold/flu season.

Fungal Infections

Depending on the type of fungal infection, combat it through internal, topical, or aromatic application, according to its location. For instance, if you have athlete's foot, topical application may be the easiest and most direct solution.

Hepatitis

Target hepatitis by steaming two drops of melaleuca essential oil in a pan of water. Then remove the steaming pan from the stove, pour into a bowl, place a towel over your head and inhale. If you don't feel it's done its job the first time, you can reheat that same water and use it once more without adding more oil. You can also dilute melaleuca in a 1:1 ratio with a carrier oil and apply topically, massaging it into the hands and the soles of the feet every day.

Herpes Simplex

Combat herpes simplex virus by diluting melaleuca in a 1:1 ratio with a carrier oil and applying topically to the affected area or massaging it into the soles of the feet every day.

Hives

Eliminate hives by diluting melaleuca in a 1:1 ratio with a carrier oil and applying topically to the affected area.

Immune Stimulant

Give your immune system a leg up by regularly diffusing melaleuca throughout your home, especially during cold and flu season. The scent also uplifts and boosts energy. Alternatively, you can add a couple drops to your bathwater or dilute with a carrier oil and apply topically, massaging it into the soles of the feet. If you'd prefer the steam method, steam two drops of melaleuca essential oil in a pan of water, remove the steaming pan from the stove, pour into a bowl, place a towel over your head and inhale. If you don't feel it's done its job the first time, you can reheat that same water and use it once more without adding more oil.

Infected Wounds

To support infected wounds, steam two drops of melaleuca essential oil in a pan of water. Then remove the steaming pan from the stove, pour into a bowl, place a towel over your head and inhale. If you don't feel it's done its job the first time, you can reheat that same water and use it once more without adding more oil. You can also diffuse or apply a single drop to warm water and soak the infected wound.

Inflammation

Calm inflammation and provide lymphatic system support by diluting 1 or 2 drops of melaleuca essential oil in a 1:1 ratio with a carrier oil, then apply topically, massaging it over the affected area towards the heart. You can also diffuse the oil or inhale directly.

Jock Itch

Relieve jock itch by diluting melaleuca in a 1:1 ratio with a carrier oil and applying topically to the affected area.

Lice

Eliminate lice by combining 3-4 drops with distilled water and soaking your patient's scalp and hair in the mixture. Also, soak any brushes or combs the infected patient used. Read this study about melaleuca's effects on head lice.

MRSA

Combat MRSA by diluting tea tree essential oil in a 1:1 ratio with a carrier oil and applying topically in a full-body massage or into the soles of the feet.

Mumps

Target mumps by diluting tea tree essential oil in a 1:1 ratio with a carrier oil and applying topically in a full-body massage or into the soles of the feet. You can also diffuse the oil throughout the home.

Nail Infection

Combine 1-2 drops of tea tree essential oil with 1 tablespoon of coconut oil and apply to cuticles and nails to combat nail infection.

Piercings

Relieve the pain from new piercings and protect against infection by diluting tea tree essential oil in a 1:1 ratio with a carrier oil and applying topically to the affected area.

Pink Eye

To relieve pink eye, steam two drops of melaleuca essential oil in a pan of water. Then remove the steaming pan from the stove, pour into a bowl, place a towel over your head and inhale, keeping your eyes open. If you don't feel it's done its job the first time, you can reheat that same water and use it once more without adding more oil.

Rashes

Rashes can be alleviated by diluting tea tree essential oil in a 1:1 ratio with a carrier oil and applying topically to the affected area.

Ringworm

Ringworm can be targeted topically by diluting tea tree essential oil with a carrier oil and massaging it over the affected area three times a day. Once the ringworm is eliminated, continue the application for 3-5 days following recovery.

Rubella

Combat rubella by diluting tea tree essential oil in a 1:1 ratio with a carrier oil and applying topically to the affected area or massaging it into the soles of the feet.

Scabies

Eliminate the mites that cause scabies, rid of the rash, and protect against infection by diluting tea tree essential oil in a 1:1 ratio with a carrier oil and applying topically to the affected area.

Shingles

Relieve and eliminate shingles by diluting melaleuca essential oil in a 1:1 ratio with a carrier oil, then apply topically, massaging over the oil over the affected area and into the soles of the feet. You can also add a few drops to a warm bath. The oil's antiviral and anti-inflammatory properties will help eliminate shingles.

Shock

Alleviate shock by diluting tea tree essential oil in a 1:1 ratio with a carrier oil, then apply topically, massaging it into the soles of your feet.

Sore Throat

Support the body's natural defenses against throat infections by diluting tea tree essential oil in a 1:1 ratio with a carrier oil and applying topically to the throat. You can also diffuse throughout the home or combine the oil with sea salts and warm water for a gargling solution.

Staph Infection

Target staph infections by diluting melaleuca essential oil with a carrier oil and massaging into the soles of the feet. This will cause your body to absorb the oil faster.

Tattoos

Stave off infections and promote healing in new tattoos by diluting melaleuca essential oil with a carrier oil and applying topically to the affected area.

Thrush

Relieve thrush with a sea salt gargle. Blend warm water, sea salt and 1 drop of tea tree oil and gargle for thirty seconds. Spit out solution.

Tonsillitis

Eliminate tonsillitis by diluting melaleuca essential oil in a 1:1 ratio with a carrier oil and applying topically into the throat and the soles of the feet. You can also diffuse throughout the home or combine the oil with sea salts and warm water for a gargling solution.

Vaginal Infection

Vaginal infections can be targeted externally. Dilute melaleuca essential oil with a carrier oil and massage into the soles of the feet. You can also place 3-4 drops in a sitz bath and soak in it for 10-15 minutes.

Viral Infections

Strengthen the body's natural defenses against viral infections by diluting melaleuca essential oil with a carrier oil and massaging into the reflex points of the feet. Or, you can also place a few drops in your bathwater, diffuse, or apply a hot compress.

Warts

To eliminate warts, dilute tea tree essential oil with a carrier oil and apply directly to the wart. Continue this application until the wart is removed.

Wounds

Disinfect wounds by adding a few drops of melaleuca essential oil to into a spray bottle filled with distilled water. Spray over the wound. You may also apply a few drops to a spritz bath and soak wound for 10-15 minutes.

Varicose Veins

Reduce the appearance of varicose veins by diluting melaleuca essential oil in a 1:1 ratio with a carrier oil and applying topically in an upwards stroke towards the heart.

Blends

Antiseptic Ointment

Ingredients

- 10 drops Lemon Essential Oil

- 20 drops Lavender Essential Oil

- 50 drops Tea Tree Essential Oil

- 1 cup Carrier Oil (Olive or Almond Oil recommended)

- 1 ½ ounces Beeswax (grated)

- ¼ tsp Vitamin E Oil

Directions

Fill a saucepan with 1 inch of water. Add the grated beeswax to a mason jar and place in the saucepan. Over low-medium heat, stir the beeswax until melted. Remove from heat. Allow the beeswax to cool slightly before mixing in remaining ingredients. Stir until well combined. Apply to wounds, cuts and stings. Shake well before each use.

Athlete's Foot or Ringworm

Ingredients

- 2 drops Tea Tree Essential Oil

- 1 drop Lavender Essential Oil

- 1 tsp Carrier Oil

Directions

To relieve athlete's foot or ringworm, place all ingredients in a bowl or jar and mix thoroughly to combine. Apply solution to the affected area with a cotton swab.

Candida Cleanse

Ingredients

- 3 drops Oregano Essential Oil

- 5 drops Melaleuca Essential Oil

- 5 drops Lemon Essential Oil

Directions

To combat candida, place all ingredients into a "00" capsule, and ingest 1 capsule twice a day for a two-week period. Leave off the application for two weeks, and then repeat.

Clarifying Head Steam

Ingredients

- 1 drop Tea Tree Essential Oil

- 1 drop Peppermint Essential Oil

- 1 drop Eucalyptus Essential Oil

Directions

Steam all oils in a pan of water, remove the steaming pan from the stove, pour into a bowl, place a towel over your head and inhale for at least five minutes, keeping your eyes shut (may sting). If you don't feel it's done its job the first time, you can reheat that same water and use it once more without adding more oil.

Colds & Flu Daytime Relief

Ingredients

- 2 drops Eucalyptus Essential Oil

- 2 drops Tea Tree Essential Oil

- 2 drops Lavender Essential Oil

- 2 drops Peppermint Essential Oil

Directions

Steam all oils in a pan of water, remove the steaming pan from the stove, pour into a bowl, place a towel over your head and inhale for three to five minutes, keeping your eyes shut (may sting). If you don't feel it's done its job the first time, you can reheat that same water and use it once more without adding more oil. You can also diffuse the combination throughout the room for a similar effect.

Gum Disease

Ingredients

- 1 drops Tea Tree Essential Oil

- 1 drop Peppermint Essential Oil

- ½ cup Distilled Water

Directions

To combat gum disease, place all ingredients into a small bottle. Place the lid on and shake well to distribute. Use as normal, swishing for 30-60 seconds. Spit out solution.

Head Lice Solution

Ingredients

- 1 Tbsp Sunflower Oil

- 2 drops Tea Tree Essential Oil

- 1 drop Lavender Essential Oil

- 1 drop Eucalyptus Essential Oil

Directions

In a small bowl or jar, combine all oils, mixing thoroughly. Massage the solution into the scalp and place a plastic shower cap over the head. Allow to sit for one hour or leave on overnight. Remove the cap and shampoo the solution out of the hair, massaging the shampoo into the scalp and hair in order to eliminate oil and grease.

Nasal Congestion

Ingredients

2 drops Tea Tree Essential Oil
2 drops Rosemary Essential Oil
4 drops Niaouli Essential Oil
1 tsp Carrier Oil

Directions

Fill the tub with warm water and pour in the oil combo, stirring the tub until evenly distributed. Breathe the vapors in as you soak in the bath for 15-20 minutes. Caution: bath water will sting if you get it in your eyes.

You can also place the same combination in a diffuser for a similar effect.

Parasitic Infections

Ingredients

- 10 drops Lemon Essential Oil

- 20 drops Lavender Essential Oil

- 50 drops Tea Tree Essential Oil

- 1 cup Carrier Oil (Olive or Almond Oil recommended)

- 1 ½ ounces Beeswax (grated)

- ¼ tsp Vitamin E Oil

Directions

Fill a saucepan with 1 inch of water. Add the grated beeswax to a mason jar and place in the saucepan. Over low-medium heat, stir the beeswax until melted. Remove from heat. Allow the beeswax to cool slightly before mixing in remaining ingredients. Stir until well combined. Apply to wounds, cuts and stings. Shake well before each use.

Shea Butter

Ingredients

- 1 tsp Lavender Essential Oil

- 1 tsp Eucalyptus Essential Oil

- 1 tsp Tea Tree Essential Oil

- 1 tsp Glycerin

- 2 cups Raw Shea

Directions

Fill a large bowl with ice water. Set aside. Place all ingredients into a pyrex dish and place the dish into the ice bath. Let cool for five minutes, then whip until creamy. Apply as needed to cracked or rough skin.

Sinus & Chest Congestion Relief

Ingredients

- 2 drops Eucalyptus Essential Oil

- 2 drops Lavender Essential Oil

- 2 drops Tea Tree Essential Oil

Directions

Steam all oils in a pan of water, remove the steaming pan from the stove, pour into a bowl, place a towel over your head and inhale for three to five minutes, keeping your eyes shut (may sting). If you don't feel it's done its job the first time, you can reheat that same water and use it once more without adding more oil.

Sinus Congestion

Ingredients

- 2 drops Eucalyptus Essential Oil

- 2 drops Tea Tree Essential Oil

- 2 drops Peppermint Essential Oil

Directions

Steam all oils in a pan of water, remove the steaming pan from the stove, pour into a bowl, place a towel over your head and inhale for three to five minutes, keeping your eyes shut (may sting). If you don't feel it's done its job the first time, you can reheat that same water and use it once more without adding more oil.

Staph Infections

Ingredients

1 drop Frankincense Essential Oil
4 drops Oregano Essential Oil
4 drops Tea Tree Essential Oil
8 ounce Water

Directions

Combine all ingredients in an 8 ounce glass of drinking water, and drink three times a day – morning, noon and night.

Sunburn

Ingredients

- 1 drop Lavender Essential Oil

- 1 drop Melaleuca Essential Oil

- 1 Tbsp Coconut Oil

Directions

To relieve sunburn, place all ingredients into a small bowl or container and blend thoroughly. Apply gently to affected area.

Uplifting Vaporizer Blend

Ingredients

- 4 drops Lemon Essential Oil

- 4 drops Bergamot Essential Oil

- 2 drops Tea Tree Essential Oil

Directions

To stabilize your mood, diffuse the oils and deeply breathe in the vapors.

Chapter 3:
Melaleuca Essential Oil Studies

Many studies have been done on essential oils to discover and prove their therapeutic qualities. In the case of the great number of melaleuca studies, many of the properties attributed to the essential oil (noted in this book and elsewhere) are quite often validated through the scientific research of accredited universities and published by accredited scientific journals. In this chapter, we'll discuss a small portion of these studies. It's important to note that research on essential oils is constant and evolving. Keep up with any recent research, as it may turn up even further valuable uses of these miracle oils.

Study 1 – Anti-inflammatory

In this study published by Biol. Pharm. Bull., the antifungal and anti-inflammatory effects of melaleuca essential oil were examined, with the following results: "The onset of oral candidiasis is accompanied by inflammatory symptoms such as pain in the tongue, edema or tissue damage and lowers the quality of life (QOL) of the patient. In a murine oral candidiasis model, the effects were studied of terpinen-4-ol (T-4-ol), one of the main constituents of tea tree oil, Melaleuca alternifolia, on inflammatory reactions...In vitro analysis of the effects of terpinen-4-ol on cytokine secretion of macrophages indicated that 800 $\mu g/mL$ of this substance significantly inhibited the cytokine production of the macrophages cultured in the presence of heat-killed C. albicans cells. Based on these findings, the role of the anti-inflammatory action of T-4-ol in its therapeutic activity against oral candidiasis was discussed."

As noted, the study examined the effect of terpenin-4-ol, a chemical component of melaleuca essential oil, on inflammatory reactions caused by oral candida strains. Candida albicans develops as yeast and filamentous cells and can potentially cause genital and oral infections. Candida albicans also increases the probability of mortality in immunocompromised individuals (cancer or AIDS patients, for instance). The study showed that terpenin-4-ol was an active combatant against Candida albicans, which demonstrates melaleuca's potential as an anti-inflammatory and antifungal and its ability in combating oral candidiasis.

Reference
http://www.ncbi.nlm.nih.gov/pubmed/23649340]

https://www.jstage.jst.go.jp/article/bpb/36/5/36_b13-00033/_pdf]

Study 2 – Skin Disease

In this study published by the AAC, the antiviral effects of melaleuca essential oil were examined, with the following results: "Molluscum contagiosum is a common childhood viral skin condition and is increasingly found as a sexually transmitted disease in adults. Current treatment options are invasive, requiring tissue destruction and attendant discomfort. A greater than 90% reduction in the number of lesions was observed in 16 of 19 children treated with TTO-I...The combination of essential oil of M. alternifolia with organically bound iodine offers a safe therapeutic alternative in the treatment of childhood molluscum."

As mentioned, molluscum contagiosum is a common viral infection of the skin, also known as water warts. The virus is contagious and is transferred through physical contact between the infected and uninfected or in touching the surface of an object with which the infected may have had contact. The disease most commonly infects children, ages 1-10. It also attacks the immunodeficient and sexually active adults. The infection can be found on any area of skin, including the arms, legs and groin. The growths may itch, leading to infection, scarring, and even eczema. If untreated, the growths can remain on the skin for up to 4 years.

This study examined 53 children, administering tea tree oil on their molluscum contagiosum growths twice daily for thirty days. The application resulted in 90% infection reduction in most of the children, indicating that melaleuca essential oil may be an effective alternative or supportive remedy when it comes to this skin disease.

Reference
http://www.ncbi.nlm.nih.gov/pubmed/22395586]

http://www.ncbi.nlm.nih.gov/pmc/articles/PMC3264233/pdf/zac909.pdf]

Study 3 – Human Anisakis Simplex

In this study published by the Biomed Research International, the insecticidal effects of melaleuca essential oil were examined, with the following results: "Nematicidal activity of Melaleuca alternifolia essential oil, commonly known as tea tree oil (TTO), was assayed in vitro against L3 larvae of Anisakis simplex... The data obtained suggest that the essential oil of Melaleuca alternifolia may have a great therapeutic potential for the treatment of human anisakiasis."

Anisakis simplex is a condition involving a parasite which can infect humans after eating fish of the Anisakis species. Those who are allergic to the immunoglobulin E, produced by the parasite, might have an allergic reaction or anaphylaxis. After ingestion, the parasitic worm attempts to enter through the intestinal wall. The worm cannot penetrate the wall, so it dies, and the body's immune system responds, surrounding the worms with immune cells. This reaction can clog the digestive tract, producing intense abdominal pain and vomiting. If the larvae are not regurgitated, they can pass into the large intestine or bowel, causing a eosinophilic granulomatous response with symptoms similar to those of Crohn's disease. This study found that melaleuca essential oil showed inhibitory activity against the parasite and so could be used in supporting the body's natural defenses against human anisakiasis.

Reference
http://www.ncbi.nlm.nih.gov/pubmed/24967378]

http://www.ncbi.nlm.nih.gov/pmc/articles/PMC4055599/pdf/BMRI2014-549510.pdf]

Study 4 – Insecticidal Properties

In this study published by the Medical and Veterinary Entomology, the insecticidal effects of melaleuca essential oil were examined, with the following results: "This study aimed to evaluate the insecticidal and repellent effects of tea tree, Melaleuca alternifolia (Myrtales: Myrtaceae), and andiroba, Carapa guianensis (Sapindales: Meliaceae), essential oils on two species of fly...Tea tree oil at a concentration of 5.0% was able to kill M. domestica with 100.0% efficacy after 12 h of exposure...It is possible to conclude that these essential oils have insecticidal and repellent effects against the species of fly used in this study."

This study tested melaleuca against the Musca domestica and the Haematobia irritans, two species of flies. The Musca domestica is the common housefly, inhabiting all corners of the globe making up 91% of all flies in human homes. The Haematobia irritans is also known as the horn fly, a bloodsucking fly which is a threat to livestock. Both fly species can carry deadly diseases. Melaleuca has been found to kill Musca domestica at 100% efficacy 12 hours after exposure and to repel Haematobia irritans at 61.6% efficacy 24 hours after exposure. In conclusion, melaleuca essential oil may be considered to have insecticidal and repellent properties against these fly species.

Reference
http://www.ncbi.nlm.nih.gov/pubmed/25171605]

http://onlinelibrary.wiley.com/doi/10.1111/mve.12078/pdf]

Study 5 – Antibacterial Properties

In this study published by Journal of Antimicrobial Chemotherapy, the antibacterial effects of melaleuca essential oil were examined, with the following results: "Thirty isolates of Pseudomonas aeruginosa, 15 isolates of Pseudomonas putida and 11 isolates of Pseudomonas fluorescens were tested for susceptibility to tea tree oil

(TTO), the essential oil of Melaleuca alternifolia, and the components terpinen-4-ol, alpha-terpineol, cineole, gamma-terpinene and rho-cymene... Pseudomonas spp. are susceptible to TTO and some of its components although they are less susceptible than many other bacteria tested previously."

This study showed that melaleuca essential oil inhibited isolates of three bacterial strains, Pseudomonas aeruginosa, Pseudomonas putida, and Pseudomonas fluorescens. Pseudomonas aeruginosa is a common bacteria found in water, soil, skin flora, and in man-made environments. The bacterium thrives on moist surfaces, and so can threaten the hospital environment by finding its home on medical equipment, like catheters, resulting in cross-infection. It is, for instance, the bacterium which causes hot-tub rash. This bacterium also attacks immunocompromised patients, infecting the urinary tract, airway, wounds, burns, and resulting in blood infections. Pseudomonas putida, on the other hand, is a comparably safe species of bacteria and not an opportunistic human pathogen, like pseudomonas aeruginosa. Though not often found in humans, pseudomonas fluorescens can attack those with compromised immune systems.

The study indicated that melaleuca essential oil is effective in combatting the cells of all three strains of bacterium, demonstrating the oil's antibacterial properties.

Reference
http://www.ncbi.nlm.nih.gov/pubmed/16735435]

http://jac.oxfordjournals.org/content/58/2/449.full.pdf+
html]

Study 6 – Influenza

In this study published by Molecules, the antiviral
effects of melaleuca essential oil were examined, with the
following results: "Influenza virus causes high morbidity
among the infected population annually and occasionally
the spread of pandemics. Melaleuca alternifolia Concentrate
(MAC) is an essential oil derived from a native Australian
tea tree. Our aim was to investigate whether MAC has any
in vitro inhibitory effect on influenza virus infection and
what mechanism does the MAC use to fight the virus
infection. In this study, the antiviral activity of MAC was
examined by its inhibition of cytopathic effects... We found
that when the influenza virus was incubated with 0.010%
MAC for one hour, no cytopathic effect on MDCK cells
was found after the virus infection and no
immunofluorescence signal was detected in the host cells.
Electron microscopy showed that the virus treated with
MAC retained its structural integrity. By computational
simulations, we found that terpinen-4-ol, which is the major
bioactive component of MAC, could combine with the
membrane fusion site of haemagglutinin. Thus, we proved
that MAC could prevent influenza virus from entering the
host cells by disturbing the normal viral membrane fusion

procedure."

This study demonstrated how melaleuca essential oil can be used to disrupt the influenza virus from entering host cells. Again, the major component indicated in this inhibitory activity was terpinen-4-ol. Melaleuca essential oil was not found to be cytopathic (it did not affect the virus' structural integrity), however, it did act as a bouncer, protecting against influenza from entering the host by interrupting the fusion of haemagglutinin, the clumping together of bacteria or red blood cells.

Reference
http://www.ncbi.nlm.nih.gov/pubmed/23966077]

Reference & Photo Credit: http://www.mdpi.com/1420-3049/18/8/9550]

Study 7 – Head Lice

In this study published by Parasitol Res, the effects melaleuca essential oil has on head lice were examined, with the following results: "Head lice infestation is an emerging social problem in undeveloped and developed countries. Because of louse resistance increasing, several long-used insecticidal compounds have lost their efficacy, and supplements, such as essential oils, have been proposed to treat this parasitic infestation. The present study investigated the efficacy of two natural substances: tea tree (Melaleuca alternifolia) oil and nerolidol (3,7,11-trimethyl-1,6,10-dodecatrien-3-ol) against lice and its eggs...Tea tree oil was more effective than nerolidol against head lice with 100 % mortality at 30 min and 1 % concentration...These results offer new potential application of natural compounds and display a promising scenario in the treatment of pediculosis resistant cases. The development of novel pediculicides containing essential oils could be, in fact, an important tool to control the parasitic infestation."

Being that the established insecticidal compounds have become ineffective due to immune resistance from long-term use, alternative methods of exterminating head lice in both developed and underdeveloped countries has been under the microscope. This study demonstrates that melaleuca could be a safe alternative. At a 1% concentration, melaleuca administration showed 100% mortality of head lice after a mere 30 minutes.

Reference
http://www.ncbi.nlm.nih.gov/pubmed/22847279]

http://www.ncbi.nlm.nih.gov/pmc/articles/PMC3480584/pdf/436_2012_Article_3045.pdf]

Study 8 – Antimicrobial Properties

In this study published by the Journal of Applied Microbiology, the antimicrobial effects of melaleuca essential oil were examined, with the following results: "The essential oil of Melaleuca alternifolia (tea tree) exhibits broad-spectrum antimicrobial activity. Its mode of action against the Gram-negative bacterium Escherichia coli AG100, the Gram-positive bacterium Staphylococcus aureus NCTC 8325, and the yeast Candida albicans has been investigated using a range of methods...We report that exposing these organisms to minimum inhibitory and minimum bactericidal/fungicidal concentrations of tea tree oil inhibited respiration and increased the permeability of bacterial cytoplasmic and yeast plasma membranes as indicated by uptake of propidium iodide. In the case of E. coli and Staph. aureus, tea tree oil also caused potassium ion leakage...The ability of tea tree oil to disrupt the permeability barrier of cell membrane structures and the accompanying loss of chemiosmotic control is the most likely source of its lethal action at minimum inhibitory levels."

Melaleuca was tested against Gram-negative bacterium Escherichia coli AG100, Gram-positive bacterium Staphylococcus aureus NCTC 8325, and the yeast Candida albicans. This study tested the antibacterial properties of melaleuca against Escherichia coli and Staphylococcus aureus, as well as against the fungi Candida albicans. Staphylococcus aureus is Gram-positive bacterium.

Although Staphylococcus aureus is part of the normal human skin flora and respiratory tract and is not typically pathogenic, those with compromised immune systems can potentially develop an infection from the bacteria. When it becomes so, S. aureus produces respiratory issues like sinusitis, skin infections, and even food poisoning. Escherichia coli is a bacterium, as well, though it's Gram negative, rather than Gram positive. E. coli can often result in serious food poisoning. Candida albicans, as described in the first study of this chapter, develops as yeast and filamentous cells and can potentially cause genital and oral infections.

Melaleuca essential showed antimicrobial activity at minimum inhibitory levels against all three strains, as the oil disrupts the permeability barrier of these cell membrane structures.

Reference
http://www.ncbi.nlm.nih.gov/pubmed/10735256]

http://onlinelibrary.wiley.com/doi/10.1046/j.1365-2672.2000.00943.x/pdf]

Chapter 4:
The Ins & Outs of Essential Oils

Where do essential oils come from?

Plants and plant species naturally produce essential oils for various reasons, one being to draw pollinator insects to them, another being to repel invading organisms (bacteria, animals). A number of chemical compounds compose each plant's essential oil, and the combination of these compounds is specific to each oil, which then instills in the oil its own unique properties. Essential oils can be harnessed from all sorts of plant components, including flowers, leaves, bark, fruit, roots, and resin. For instance, cinnamon oil is harnessed from bark, lemon oil from the peel, and lavender oil from lavender flowers. Certain plants can produce a few chemical variants of the same essential oil, which are acquired from different parts of the plant. Some of these parts produce a large amount of oil, while others produce just a smidgen. The oil's quality and potency depends upon a number of factors, including the subspecies of the plant, its soil conditions, the time of year and even the time of day you harvest it.

How are essential oils extracted?

Essential oils can be extracted from plants through various methods, including pressing, distillation, solvent and maceration. Let's take a brief look at each:

Pressing Method

Commonly used with citrus fruit, the pressing method extracts the oil through a technique which involves pushing the fruit peels through a press. Oily fruits and plants are best suited for this technique. Orange oil, for example, is extracted from orange skins through the pressing method.

Distillation Method

This technique harkens back to the days of old-timey moonshiners, as the same sort of method used to create strong liquor can be used to extract essential oils. Using a still, boiled water and plant materials will create steam which is then cooled by coils and condensed into a combination of water and oil. This combination doesn't mix, so the oil can then be extracted from it.

Solvent Method

Through a multi-step process, certain plant and flower oils can be extracted using alcohol and other solvents, which extort the essential oil from the plant materials.

Maceration Method

When a "carrier" or fixed oil or lard is mixed with the plant material and set out in the sun, over a period of time, the carrier oil is infused with the plant's essence. Heat sources, other than the sun, are often used to speed the process. Throughout the process, more plant material is added to produce a more potent oil.

How do you use essential oils?

Although some studies about the effectiveness of essential oils are conducted by small companies or even individuals, a number of them are conducted by the food and cosmetic industries. In general, the pharmaceutical industry shows next to no interest in herbal medicine, primarily because there are few options to patent such products. Being as such, the product's lack of profitability results in a lack of research funding. Regardless, the historical uses of essential oils tell us what we need to know: these oils have been effectively administered for centuries. The therapeutic qualifications of essential oils can be plotted in the survival of the human race across cultures and generations.

Another reason that studies on essential oils have not resulted in much conclusive evidence as to their overall effectiveness is because definitive results are sometimes difficult to prove, as the quality of each batch of oil can vary for a number of reasons. One is that essential oils are impossible to standardize. As mentioned above, even the slightest variance in soil conditions and the time of harvesting – as well as innumerable other factors – will produce a different product quality and potency. In addition, essential oils are often obtained from various species of the same plant; Eucalyptus radiata and Eucalyptus globulus can both be used in the making of therapeutic-grade eucalyptus oil and, as a result, they may have slightly different properties and degrees of strength or effectiveness.

Just as there are a number of methods by which to extract essential oils, there are a number of methods to administer them therapeutically. The variety of chemical compounds in each essential oil means that their benefits and applications also vary across the board. Below are a few of these methods.

Topical Administration

Direct application of many essential oils works like a sponge, as skin sops up chemicals and other things (like sunlight, for instance). Topical application is best when you want to clear up an ailment on the skin's surface or in the underlying muscle tissue. When applying topically, you may either massage the oil into the skin or simply dab on the skin for therapeutic results. You might combine the essential oil with a carrier oil for topical use in order to dilute its potency. This is safer, as the oil is so concentrated. You may support your body's defenses against rash or muscle pain in this manner, but you should always test your patient for allergies before applying. Adverse effects are produced by natural chemicals as much as synthetic ones; poison ivy, for example.

To test for allergens, place a drop or two on your patient's inner forearm. If a rash develops within 12 to 24 hours, then the patient is allergic. In addition, phototoxicity – sun exposure resulting in an exacerbated burn – may be an issue when citrus oils are applied topically. So one must proceed with caution when applying essential oils using this method.

Inhalation Therapy

Commonly known as "aromatherapy", this essential oil application is effective for inner ailments, like sore throat or cold. In a steaming bowl of distilled or sterilized water, add a few drops of essential oil and, with a towel over your head, bend over the bowl and inhale. The towel captures the vapors, making the technique even more effective. Essential oils can also be placed in a diffuser or potpourri throughout a room to produce somewhat diluted therapeutic effects.

Ingestion

When using this method, proceed with caution. Direct ingestion of essential oils must be monitored and applied in small doses that are diluted in a tablespoon or more of any carrier oil – olive oil, for example. If you are unsure of dosage amounts, make a tea with the relevant herb instead. Although the effects of this diluted use may be weaker, this application is a better alternative than an overdose of essential oils.

What are the general benefits of using essential oils?

Replacement for Prescription Drugs

One practical benefit for using essential oils is, of course, their substitutive nature; they can replace Rx drugs, which is the ultimate reason to educate yourself on their administration and to begin stockpiling your essential oil supply. One of the potential threats of economic or social collapse is the lack of resources, and primarily the inability to procure prescription drugs. Being as such, finding suitable supplements should be a priority when preparing for the worst.

Their portability is also a major bonus when it comes to survival prepping. The fact that these ultra-concentrated oils take up little-to-no space makes toting them to your shelter all the simpler should the need arise. And, because essential oils are highly concentrated, the application used in most methods of administration requires only a drop or two of oil, which means that tiny bottle will be long-lasting.

Cost Effective Supplement

Though money may be the last thing on your mind when it comes to prepping for a survival situation (money may even be obsolete in the event of social collapse), it is worth noting that the expense of essential oils pales in comparison to prescription drugs. Essential oils are a cost effective supplement to prescription medicine.

No Expiration Date

Another benefit of essential oils is that they do not expire, neither do they have "proper storage" requirements. A number of medicines and medicinal products must be replaced every couple years, so this sets essential oils ahead of the pack when it comes to shelf life.

Versatility

Essential oils also offer great versatility. Apart from providing therapeutic benefits, essential oils can be repurposed for household and hygienic applications. For instance, if you're looking for something that might serve your dental hygiene needs in a time of crisis, the protective oil blend is your go-to essential oil. If you want to maintain your skin's tone and condition, frankincense and lavender will do the trick; the latter also serves as sunscreen, so you can inhibit sun damage as well.

When it comes to the house or shelter, you can use essential oils to deodorize, which will come in handy in a disaster scenario where things might start to smell fishy due to lack of proper utilities and care. For example, after the 2011 tsunami and the subsequent nuclear reactor meltdown in Japan, a nurse named Risa Nakahira used essential oils to deodorize and sanitize putrid public bathrooms in overpopulated evacuation facilities. As relief workers searched for survivors, often wading through debris and decay, Nakahira also deodorized their boots and masks using essential oils. The possibilities of these natural oils are endless.

They are also versatile when it comes to the range of patients they're capable of supporting. The wellness of everyone from your great grandfather to your infant baby can be fortified with the aid of essential oils in the appropriate dosage. They even come in handy when supporting the wellness of livestock or pets. From teething infants to dementia in the elderly, from teenagers with acne to dogs with urinary tract infections, essential oils can serve any patient with nearly any ailment.

Conclusion

Now that you know all about what melaleuca essential oil can do for you – where it originates, how it's extracted, its benefits and properties, and the different methods of administration – you can use it confidently to support the body's defenses against wellness issues and start to assemble a kit of essential oils for survival. Essential oils can be purchased online or at your local holistic treatment store. We always recommend the brand guarantees high quality therapeutic grade oils and carries a certification of third party testing.

The various benefits of essential oils and their properties are countless. To build your own kit, first focus on acquiring the essential oils which may bear more relevance to your wellness issues or the potential threats within your environment. In the event of a viral outbreak, for instance, melaleuca essential oil will be one of your more crucial oils – along with oregano, lemon, frankincense and cinnamon (eBooks also available for purchase) – due to their antiviral and immuno-supportive properties.

Used as a supplement or as your go-to for skin issues, viral infections or immune-boosting agents, the application of melaleuca essential oil in medicine has survived for centuries and will survive centuries more. When it comes down to it, you don't need to rely on pharmaceuticals; essential oils, herbs, and plenty of other natural ingredients can be used to help support the body's natural defenses against any number of wellness issues, whether ailment or injury.

Essential oils are essential to your survival in the case of viral outbreak, social collapse or natural disaster because, when the SHTF, your access to pharmaceuticals will likely either be limited or eliminated altogether. Supplements to our modern-day standard will equate survival when no other option exists. And when it comes to a life-or-death situation, you can't let your wellness decline, no matter the state of the world.

DISCLAIMER AND/OR LEGAL NOTICES: Every effort has been made to accurately represent this book and it's potential. Results vary with every individual, and your results may or may not be different from those depicted. No promises, guarantees or warranties, whether stated or implied, have been made that you will produce any specific result from this book. Your efforts are individual and unique, and may vary from those shown. Your success depends on your efforts, background and motivation.

The material in this publication is provided for educational and informational purposes only and is not intended as medical advice. The information contained in this book should not be used to diagnose or treat any illness, metabolic disorder, disease or health problem. Always consult your physician or healthcare provider before beginning any nutrition or exercise program. Use of the programs, advice, and information contained in this book is at the sole choice and risk of the reader.